THE AMAZING
WATER BOTTLE
WORKOUT

NO GYM? NO WEIGHTS? NO PROBLEM!

T0273534

BY JASON S. GREENSPAN AND LEE NOONAN

The information contained in this book is based upon the personal and professional experiences of the authors. It is not intended as a substitute for consulting with your physician or other healthcare provider. Prior to beginning any exercise program, it is recommended that you consult your physician.

The publisher does not advocate the use of any particular exercise protocol but believes the information in this book should be available to the public. The publisher and authors are not responsible for any adverse effects or consequences resulting from the use of the suggestions, techniques, or procedures discussed in this book. Should the reader have any questions concerning the appropriateness of any exercise regimen mentioned, the authors and the publisher strongly suggest consulting a professional healthcare advisor.

Basic Health Publications, Inc.
28812 Top of the World Drive
Laguna Beach, CA 92651
949-715-7327 • www.basichealthpub.com

Library of Congress Cataloging-in-Publication Data

Greenspan, Jason S.
    The amazing water bottle workout : No gym? No weights? No problem! /
Jason S. Greenspan and Lee Noonan.
        p. cm.
    Includes bibliographical references and index.
    ISBN 978-1-59120-281-3
    1. Weight lifting. 2. Water bottles. 3. Physical fitness. I. Noonan, Lee II. Title.
    GV546.3.G74   2010
    613.7'13—dc22

                                                            2010004337

Design by WestGroup Creative • www.westgp.com
Photography by Eric Goldstein
Models: Sharon Forman and Edward Marks

Printed in the United States of America

10   9   8   7   6   5   4   3   2   1

CONTENTS

INTRODUCTION

You may laugh when you think of using water bottles to increase strength, but think again. Water is heavy and, like dumbbells, water bottles come in different shapes and sizes. Best of all, they are available EVERYWHERE! You don't need a gym. You don't need weights or elastic bands. You just need to understand the true power of water.

Water in bottles is just another form of resistance. When you exercise, your muscles aren't aware of the source of the resistance. It could be dumbbells, elastic bands, machines, a big rock… or bottles filled with water.

Still laughing? Consider all the following reasons a water bottle workout is a smart, effective way to get fit.

- **Convenient:** you don't need a gym or gym equipment;
- **Time-Saving:** no need to travel to an exercise location;
- **Accessible:** water bottles can be purchased almost anywhere;
- **Portable:** perfect for workouts at home, in the office or hotel room;
- **Stabilizing:** like dumbbells, water bottles require you to use stabilizing muscles to balance and control the weight.

The Amazing the Water Bottle Workout is:

- **Thorough:** these carefully-conceived workouts address the entire body and are geared for every fitness level;
- **Challenging:** though water bottles have weight limitations, we offer time and balance challenges to further test your strength and endurance;
- **Practical:** bottles of water are inexpensive; then you can drink the water!
- **Green:** environmentally-friendly stainless steel water bottles can be substituted for plastic ones.

There are no more excuses for not working out. YOU can get fit and have fun doing it without joining a gym. No one will be watching, judging, intimidating you and your efforts to succeed. You can exercise at home, at work, on vacation, on business trips . . . any and everywhere.

Grab those water bottles and let's get started!

 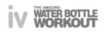

If you feel any discomfort while doing these exercises or suggested modifications, immediately stop your workout and consult a physician.

GUIDELINES

- Consult a physician before beginning a new workout program.
- Warm up prior to exercising.
- Work the larger muscles first (lower body), progressing to the smaller muscles; then work the core.
- Stretch after working out.
- Exhale when lifting water bottles (or upon exertion). Never hold your breath.
- Work within your comfortable (pain-free) range of motion.
- Lift water bottles in a controlled manner to eliminate momentum.
- Maintain proper posture throughout each exercise.

DETERMINE YOUR FITNESS LEVEL
Before you begin the water bottle exercises, you will need to determine your fitness level.

Beginner: working out for less than 6 months using light-to-moderate weights and doing a moderate volume of exercises; experienced mostly with machines.

Intermediate: working out for 8 months to 1 year using medium-to-heavy weights and doing a greater volume of exercises; experienced with free weights.

Advanced: working out on a regular basis for at least 1 year with heavy weights, doing a high volume of exercises; experienced with free weights.

SELECT YOUR WATER BOTTLE WEIGHTS
See page viii to understand the best water bottle weight for your fitness level.

BEST RESULTS

To get the best results from *The Amazing Water Bottle Workout*, we suggest the following strategies:

- *before* doing any workout, review every exercise in this book;
- find the variation and form of each exercise that best matches your fitness level;
- choose one of the four workouts on pages 19–23;
- follow the exact order of a particular circuit;
- pay attention to suggested rep cycles and sets.

PROGRESSIONS/CHALLENGES

- When you are comfortable with completing 15 reps, progress by increasing the water bottle weight;
- The second challenge is to slow down the movement from a traditional 6 second repetition to a 10 second rep cycle, eliminating momentum;
- Then try doing all of the above on one leg to engage the core.

NOTE: In addition to the workouts in this book, we suggest that you participate in a cardiovascular program 3–5 days/week, working up to 30 minutes per day. You may use one or more of the warm-up exercises on page vii to create a program for yourself.

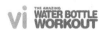

WARM-UP

The crucial warm-up period increases body temperature. Warmer muscles move more freely and with greater ease.

Duration: 5–10 minutes prior to working out, using any combination of the following suggested forms.

BEGINNER WARM-UP

Speed-walk around the room or up and down a hallway for 5 minutes. Hold elbows at 90° and pump arms while walking.

INTERMEDIATE WARM-UP

Climb stairs—up and down—for 5 minutes, with elbows at 90°. Pace your exertion with your current endurance level.

Jog in place for 5 minutes. Hold elbows at 90° and pump arms while jogging.

ADVANCED WARM-UP

Jumping rope (if no rope, simulate movement) for 5 minutes. Jumping rope quickly burns calories and tones muscles. May be done with a skipping or jumping motion.

Shadow-box for 5 minutes while keeping feet in motion. Increases heart rate quickly; moves lots of muscles simultaneously.

GLOSSARY OF ABBREVIATIONS

Rep(s) = repetition(s)

WB(s) = water bottle(s)

BEG = beginner

INT = intermediate

ADV = advanced

Sec(s) = second(s)

ROM = range of motion

SP = starting position

Abs = abdominal muscles

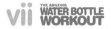

THE AMAZING
WATER BOTTLE
WORKOUT

WATER BOTTLE SELECTION

You can purchase bottles of water in a variety of sizes and shapes in most food and convenience stores. When selecting your bottles, think of both the shape (for easy gripping) and the weight. Many exercises require two water bottles of the same weight. Some exercises use one heavier water bottle.

WEIGHT SELECTION

Pick a weight you can comfortably use to complete at least 10 repetitions of an exercise. Once you can easily achieve 15 reps, it is time to increase the weight of your water bottle. This concept of progressive resistance should continue as you improve your strength and endurance.

BEGINNER: Smaller bottles are most appropriate (3–6 lbs)

INTERMEDIATE/ADVANCED: Heavier bottles (9–22 lbs)

WEIGHT EQUIVALENTS

Plastic Water Bottles

1 liter = 3 lb

1.5 liter = 4 lb

2.2 liter = 5 lb

3 liter= 6 lb

1 gallon = 9 lb

2.5 gallon = 22 lb

Stainless Steel Water Bottles

27 oz = 1 lb

40 oz = 3 lb

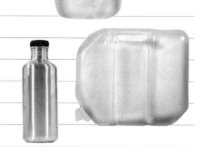

GREEN ALTERNATIVES: For those who dislike plastic water bottles, you can find non-plastic alternatives on the Internet or in stores that sell environmentally-friendly items. We like the stainless steel bottles that are washable and reusable. They come in a variety of sizes and shapes.

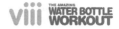

EXERCISES

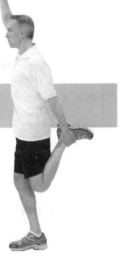

HISTORY OF KNEE PROBLEMS?
*When doing squats—or any exercise—ALWAYS work within your pain-free
ROM. If the Standard Squat is uncomfortable, bend knees only slightly.
If still uncomfortable SKIP THESE EXERCISES.*

STANDARD SQUAT 2 WATER BOTTLES—ALL LEVELS

STARTING POSITION

- Stand with feet shoulder width apart, toes point slightly outward (30°).
- Arms at sides, palms face thighs, each holds a WB.

POSTURE: Abs tight, chest lifted, shoulders down and back,
eyes straight ahead.

TIMING: 6 sec reps: 4 secs down, 2 secs up.

PROPER FORM

1 Inhale. Drop hips backwards as if sitting, while bending both knees.

2 Maintain proper posture, lower thighs until parallel to ground.

3 Keep knees over ankles, pointing toward toes.

4 Exhale. Push up through heels until legs are straight, knees unlocked.

COMMON MISTAKES

- *Rounding back, lifting heels, looking down.*
- *Moving knees beyond toes.*
- *Letting knees buckle in or out.*
- *Allowing buttocks to go lower than knees.*

- Strengthening muscles
- Stabilizing the knee joint
- Creating a firm foundation

Daily activities become easier and sports performance is enhanced.

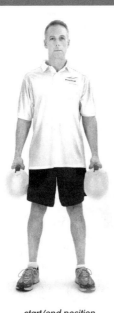

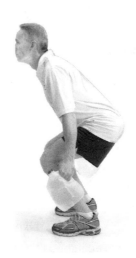

start/end position   *mid-point position*

BEGINNERS
- Start with back against a wall for support, keep contact with wall at all times.

INTERMEDIATE PROGRESSION
- Increase intensity by increasing weight.

ADVANCED CHALLENGES
- 10 sec reps—6 secs down, 4 secs up.
- Extra Challenge: **ONE-LEGGED SQUAT**.
  - Change starting position to one leg on floor, other knee is slightly bent and lifted off floor.
  - Follow proper form (see above).

PLIÉ SQUAT 2 WATER BOTTLESALL LEVELS

STARTING POSITION

- Stand with feet wider than shoulder width.
- Toes point at a 45° angle.
- Hold 1 WB between thighs with hands.

POSTURE: Abs tight, chest lifted, shoulders down and back, eyes straight ahead.

TIMING: 6 sec reps: 4 secs down, 2 secs up.

PROPER FORM

1 Inhale. Bend both knees, keeping back straight.

2 Maintain proper posture, lower thighs until parallel to ground.

3 Keep knees over ankles, pointing toward toes.

4 Exhale. Push up through heels until legs are straight, knees unlocked.

COMMON MISTAKES

- *Rounding back, lifting heels, looking down.*
- *Moving knees beyond toes.*
- *Letting knees buckle in or out.*
- *Allowing buttocks to go lower than knees.*

 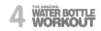

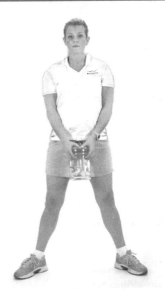

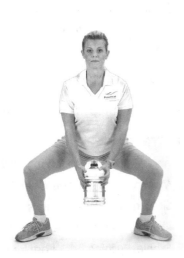

start/end position   *mid-point position*

BEGINNERS
- Start with back against a wall for support, keep contact with wall at all times.

INTERMEDIATE PROGRESSION
- Increase intensity by increasing weight.

ADVANCED CHALLENGES
- 10 sec reps: 6 secs down, 4 secs up.
- Extra Challenge: 10 seconds down, hold 2 seconds, 10 seconds up.

ALTERNATING LUNGE 2 WATER BOTTLES—INT/ADVANCED LEVEL

STARTING POSITION
- Stand with feet shoulder width apart, toes straight ahead.
- Arms at sides of thighs, each holds 1 WB.

POSTURE: Abs tight, chest lifted, shoulders down and back, eyes straight ahead.

TIMING: 6 sec reps: 2 secs forward, 4 secs back.

PROPER FORM
1 Inhale. Take a long step forward with left leg.
2 Maintain proper posture and keep hips under shoulders.
3 Simultaneously bend knees to create 90° angles.
4 Right heel lifts, left knee over ankle, pointing at toes.
5 Exhale. Pushing back from front heel, straighten both knees, bringing front foot to SP.
6 Repeat steps 1–5 using right leg.

COMMON MISTAKES
- *Rounding back, looking down.*
- *Moving front knee beyond toes.*
- *Letting front knee buckle in or out.*
- *Allowing back knee to touch ground.*

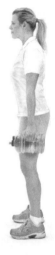 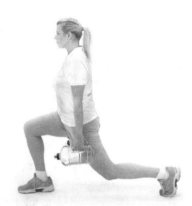

start/end position   *mid-point position*

BEGINNERS: STATIONARY LUNGE
- Eliminate form step 5.
- Keeping hips under shoulders, raise and lower body straight up and straight down.
- If needed for balance, hold wall with one hand.
- Change forward leg and repeat.

INTERMEDIATE PROGRESSION
- Increase intensity by increasing weight.

ADVANCED CHALLENGE: WALKING LUNGE WITH ROTATION
- Hold one larger WB in both hands chest high.
- As you step forward with left leg, rotate torso to left.
- Rotate torso back to center, then take a long step forward with rear leg as you rotate torso to right.
- Rotate torso back to center and continue lunging.

 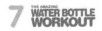

CAUTION! HISTORY OF LOWER BACK PAIN? SKIP THIS EXERCISE.

DEADLIFT 2 WATER BOTTLES—ALL LEVELS

STARTING POSITION:

- Feet shoulder width apart, toes straight ahead.
- Knees soft (not bent, not straight).
- Arms relaxed, palms face front of thighs, holding WBs.

POSTURE: Abs tight, chest lifted, shoulders down and back, eyes straight ahead.

TIMING: 6 sec reps: 4 secs down, 2 secs up.

PROPER FORM

1 Inhale. Bend forward from the hip while pushing buttocks to the rear.

2 Water bottles are close to thigh and knees are soft.

3 Keeping back flat, continue to lower WBs to mid- shin level or within your comfort zone.

4 Exhale. Push up through heels and pull up through the back of the leg as you rise to SP.

COMMON MISTAKES

- *Bending knees on descent.*
- *Locking knees when rising.*
- *Rounding back, looking down.*
- *Allowing WBs to stray away from thighs.*

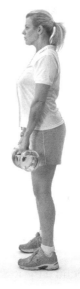
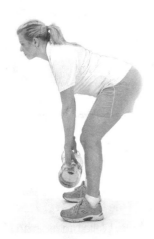

start/end position   *mid-point position*

BEGINNERS
- Modify movement by only lowering WBs to top of knees.
  Return to SP.

INTERMEDIATE PROGRESSION
- Increase intensity by increasing weight.

ADVANCED CHALLENGE: ONE-LEGGED DEADLIFT
- Stand on one foot, bend other knee slightly and raise leg.
- Follow form steps 1–4.
- Change legs and repeat.

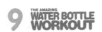

SEATED ROW 2 WATER BOTTLES—BEGINNER LEVEL

STARTING POSITION

- Sit at the edge of a chair, feet flat on floor, shoulder width apart.
- Arms extend forward at chest level, palms facing each other.
- Each hand holds a WB.

POSTURE: Abs tight, chest lifted, shoulders down and back, eyes straight ahead.

TIMING: 6 sec reps: 2 secs drawing elbows up, 4 secs return.

PROPER FORM

1 Exhale as you draw shoulder blades toward each other.
2 Keeping elbows close to sides, pull WBs back until elbows are just past the torso.
3 Inhale. While maintaining shoulder position, extend arms to SP.

COMMON MISTAKES

- *Rounding back, lifting shoulders.*
- *Allowing elbows to leave sides.*
- *Letting WBs rise above chest level.*

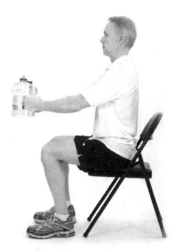

start/end position

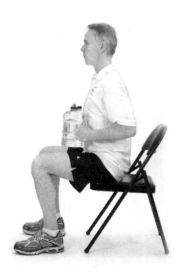

mid-point position

ONE-ARMED ROW 1 WATER BOTTLE—BEG/INT LEVELS

STARTING POSITION

- Kneel with right knee in center of a cushioned chair.
- Left leg on floor, knee at same level as other knee and slightly bent.
- Right hand rests on chair directly under right shoulder.
- Left arm is fully extended and slightly forward.
- Left hand holds WB with palm facing inward, in line with non-working hand.

POSTURE: Back is flat and parallel to ground.

TIMING: 6 sec reps: 2 secs drawing elbow up, 4 secs return.

PROPER FORM

1 Exhale. Keeping left elbow close to body, bend arm as you draw WB up until even with torso.
2 Inhale. Lower WB and return to SP.
3 Place left knee on chair and lift WB with right arm.
4 Movement is like sawing wood.

COMMON MISTAKES

- *Allowing elbow to stray from side of body during any phase of motion.*
- *Rotating torso; rounding back.*
- *Shrugging shoulders.*

- **Helps improve posture**
- **Stabilizes the shoulder**

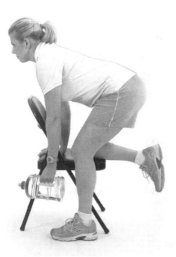

start/end position

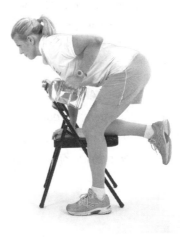

mid-point position

HISTORY OF LOWER BACK PAIN?
Do the ONE-ARMED ROW on page 13.

BENT OVER ROW 2 WATER BOTTLES—ADVANCED LEVEL

STARTING POSITION

- Feet shoulder width apart, toes straight ahead.
- Bend forward from hip until back is parallel—or just above parallel—to the floor.
- Knees are slightly bent, arms extended at sides, palms facing each other, each hand holds a WB.

POSTURE: Abs tight, chest lifted, shoulders down and back, eyes straight ahead.

TIMING: 6 sec reps: 2 secs drawing elbows up, 4 secs return.

PROPER FORM

1 Exhale. Draw shoulder blades toward each other.
2 Keeping elbows close to sides, draw WBs up until elbows are just above the level of the back.
3 Inhale. Lower WBs to SP.

COMMON MISTAKES

- *Lifting shoulders, rounding back.*
- *Allowing elbows to leave sides.*
- *Changing position of back, locking knees.*

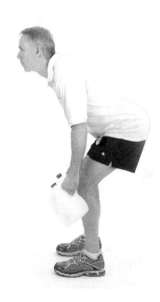

start/end position

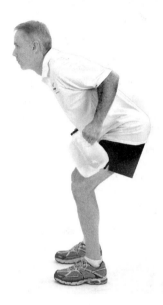

mid-point position

ADVANCED CHALLENGE: ONE-LEGGED ROW
- Stand on one foot, bend other knee slightly and raise leg.
- Follow form steps 1–3.
- Change legs and repeat.

HISTORY OF SHOULDER PAIN?
Decrease weight and/or change palms to
neutral position facing each other.

CHEST PRESS 2 WATER BOTTLES—ALL LEVELS

STARTING POSITION

- Lie on back on a mat or cushioned floor.
- Knees are bent, feet flat on floor.
- Arms are extended above center of chest, each hand holds a WB, palms face forward, elbows are soft (not bent, not straight).

POSTURE: Abs tight, lower back in contact with floor, shoulders down and back.

TIMING: 6 sec reps: 4 secs down, 2 secs up.

PROPER FORM

1 Inhale. Lower WBs as elbows bend out to sides.
2 Continue lowering until elbows and upper arm are in contact with floor.
3 Exhale. Keeping shoulder blades drawn together, raise WBs in slight arcing motion and return to SP.

COMMON MISTAKES

- *Arching back.*
- *Lifting hips or shoulders.*

DIFFICULTY LYING ON YOUR BACK?
Sit in a chair with back support, holding one WB in both hands at chest height. Squeeze WB as you push bottle forward until elbows are slightly bent. Return to starting position.

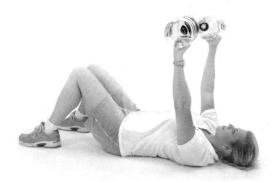

start/end position

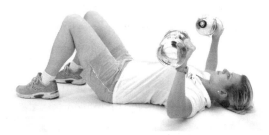

mid-point position

INTERMEDIATE PROGRESSION
- Increase intensity by increasing weight.

ADVANCED CHALLENGE
- Slower speed: 10 sec reps: 6 secs down, 4 secs up.

HISTORY OF SHOULDER PAIN?
Decrease weight and/or limit ROM by lowering WBs only halfway.

CHEST FLY 2 WATER BOTTLES—ALL LEVELS

STARTING POSITION

- Lie on back on a mat or cushioned floor.
- Knees are bent, feet flat on floor.
- Palms face each other, holding WBs directly over center of chest, elbows slightly bent.

POSTURE: Abs tight, lower back in contact with floor, shoulders down and back.

TIMING: 6 sec reps: 4 secs down, 2 secs up.

PROPER FORM

1 Inhale. Maintaining slight bend at elbows, lower WBs down and out to sides, stopping just before touching floor.

2 Elbows and shoulders stay in one line.

3 Shoulder blades stay drawn together, lower back in contact with floor.

4 Exhale. Raise WBs in semi-circular motion to SP.

5 Exercise resembles hugging motion.

COMMON MISTAKES

- *Raising hips.*
- *Straightening elbows.*
- *Collapsing elbows at lowest point.*

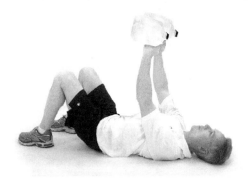

start/end position

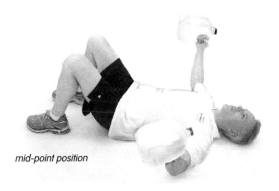

mid-point position

HINT: SUBTLE DIFFERENCE BETWEEN CHEST PRESS AND CHEST FLY—
  Chest Press = angular form
  Chest Fly = rounded form

INTERMEDIATE PROGRESSION
• Increase intensity by increasing weight.

ADVANCED CHALLENGE
• Slower speed—10 sec reps: 6 secs down, 4 secs up.

PULLOVER 1 WATER BOTTLE—ALL LEVELS

STARTING POSITION

- Lie on back on a mat or cushioned floor
- Knees are bent, feet flat on floor.
- Interlock fingers to firmly hold WB above center of chest.
- Elbows are slightly bent.

POSTURE: Abs tight, lower back in contact with floor, shoulders down and back.

TIMING: 6 sec reps: 4 secs down, 2 secs up.

PROPER FORM

1 Inhale. Maintaining slight bend at elbows, lower WB overhead until upper arms are parallel with floor.
2 Exhale. Raise WB to SP.

COMMON MISTAKES

- *Bending or straightening elbows throughout movement.*
- *Arching lower back; shrugging shoulders.*

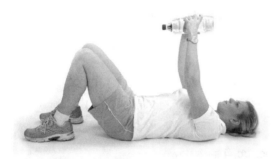

start/end position

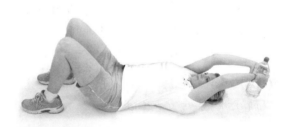

mid-point position

INTERMEDIATE PROGRESSION
• Increase intensity by increasing weight.

ADVANCED CHALLENGE
• Slower speed—10 sec reps: 6 secs down, 4 secs up.

HISTORY OF SHOULDER PAIN?
Decrease weight and/or change palms to
neutral position facing each other. Follow form steps 1–4.

SEATED SHOULDER PRESS 2 WATER BOTTLES—ALL LEVELS

STARTING POSITION

- Sit in a chair with back support, feet flat on floor, shoulder width apart.
- Arms form a 90° angle between elbow and shoulder.
- Palms face forward, holding WBs.

POSTURE: ABs tight, chest lifted, shoulders down and back, eyes straight ahead.

TIMING: 6 sec reps: 2 secs up, 4 secs down.

PROPER FORM

1 Exhale. Using an arcing motion, extend elbows and raise WBs until they almost touch.

2 WBs should be positioned slightly in front of the head.

3 Elbows are soft (not bent, not straight).

4 Inhale. Lower WBs to SP.

COMMON MISTAKES

- *Lifting shoulders, rounding back.*
- *Locking elbows.*
- *Lifting WBs directly overhead.*

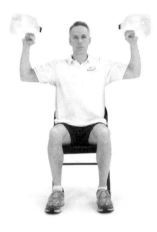

start/end position

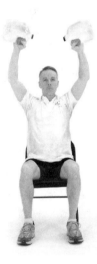

mid-point position

INTERMEDIATE PROGRESSION
- Increase intensity by increasing weight.

ADVANCED CHALLENGE: ONE-LEGGED STANDING SHOULDER PRESS
- Stand on one foot, bend other knee slightly and raise leg.
- Repeat form steps 1–4.
- Change legs and repeat.

HISTORY OF SHOULDER PAIN?
Decrease weight and/or limit ROM by keeping
WBs below shoulder level.

LATERAL RAISE 2 WATER BOTTLES—ALL LEVELS

STARTING POSITION

- Stand with feet shoulder width apart, knees slightly bent.
- Arms rest at sides of thighs, elbows slightly bent.
- Palms face legs, holding WBs.

POSTURE: Abs tight, chest lifted, shoulders down and back, eyes straight ahead.

TIMING: 6 sec reps: 2 secs up, 4 secs down.

PROPER FORM

1 Exhale. Initiating movement with elbows, raise WBs to shoulder height.

2 Inhale. Lower WBs to SP.

COMMON MISTAKES

- *Shrugging shoulders; straightening elbows.*
- *Swinging upper body.*
- *Lifting WBs above shoulder height.*

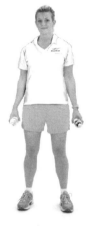

start/end position

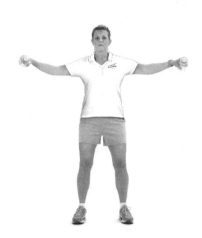

mid-point position

INTERMEDIATE PROGRESSION
- Increase intensity by increasing weight.

ADVANCED CHALLENGE: ONE-LEGGED LATERAL RAISE
- Stand on one foot, bend other knee slightly and raise leg.
- Repeat form steps 1–2.
- Change legs and repeat.

CAUTION! HISTORY OF SHOULDER PAIN? SKIP THIS EXERCISE.

UPRIGHT ROW 2 WATER BOTTLES—ALL LEVELS

STARTING POSITION

- Stand with feet shoulder width apart, knees slightly bent.
- Arms rest at front of thighs, palms face legs, holding WBs.

POSTURE: Abs tight, chest lifted, shoulders down and back, eyes straight ahead.

TIMING: 6 sec reps: 2 secs up, 4 secs down.

PROPER FORM

1 Exhale. Initiating movement with elbows, bend arms and raise WBs to shoulder height.

2 Inhale. Lower WBs to SP.

3 Always keep WBs close to body during all phases of motion.

COMMON MISTAKES

- *Shrugging shoulders.*
- *Swinging upper body.*
- *Lifting elbows above shoulders.*
- *Allowing WBs to move away from body.*

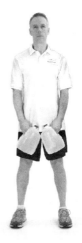

start/end position

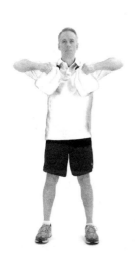

mid-point position

INTERMEDIATE PROGRESSION
• Increase intensity by increasing weight.

ADVANCED CHALLENGE: ONE-LEGGED UPRIGHT ROW
• Stand on one foot, bend other knee slightly and raise leg.
• Repeat form steps 1–3.
• Change legs and repeat.

HISTORY OF SHOULDER PAIN?
Decrease weight and/or limit ROM by keeping
WBs below shoulder level.

ALTERNATING FRONT RAISE 2 WATER BOTTLES—ALL LEVELS

STARTING POSITION

- Stand with feet shoulder width apart, knees slightly bent.
- Arms rest at front of thighs, palms face legs, holding WBs.

POSTURE: Abs tight, chest lifted, shoulders down and back, eyes straight ahead.

TIMING: 6 sec reps: 2 secs up, 4 secs down.

PROPER FORM

1 Exhale. Maintaining slight bend at elbow, raise one WB to shoulder height.

2 Inhale. Lower WB to SP.

3 Repeat with opposite arm.

COMMON MISTAKES

- *Changing angle of elbow.*
- *Shrugging shoulders.*
- *Swinging upper body.*
- *Lifting WB above shoulder height.*

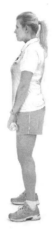

start/end position

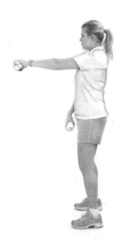

mid-point position

INTERMEDIATE PROGRESSION
- Increase intensity by increasing weight.

ADVANCED CHALLENGE: ONE-LEGGED DUAL FRONT RAISE
- Stand on one foot, bend other knee slightly and raise leg.
- Exhale. Maintaining slight bend at elbow, raise both WBs to shoulder height.
- Inhale. Lower WBs to SP.
- Change legs and repeat.

HISTORY OF SHOULDER PAIN?
Decrease weight and/or modify ROM, or skip this exercise.
HISTORY OF LOWER BACK PAIN? Change SP to sitting in a chair with
back support. Follow form steps 1–3.

OVERHEAD EXTENSION 1 WATER BOTTLE—ALL LEVELS

STARTING POSITION

- Stand with feet shoulder width apart, knees slightly bent.
- With upper arms close to ears, hold 1 WB overhead, fingers interlaced.
- Elbows are soft (not bent, not straight).

POSTURE: Abs tight, chest lifted, shoulders down and back, eyes straight ahead.

TIMING: 6 sec reps: 4 secs down, 2 secs up.

PROPER FORM

1 Inhale. Lower WB to point where elbows and shoulders form a 90° angle.
2 Exhale and return to SP.
3 Keep elbows close to head during all phases of motion.

COMMON MISTAKES

- *Elbows wandering from sides of head.*
- *Shrugging shoulders; swinging upper body.*
- *Lowering WB past 90° at elbow.*

- Strengthens and firms back of upper arm
- Increases ability to carry and to push (e.g. open a door)

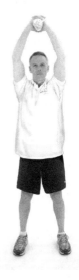

start/end position

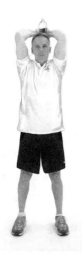

mid-point position

INTERMEDIATE PROGRESSION
- Increase intensity by increasing weight.

ADVANCED CHALLENGE
- Slower speed—10 sec reps: 6 secs down, 4 secs up.

ADVANCED BALANCE CHALLENGE
- Do exercise on one leg, change legs.

HISTORY OF LOWER BACK PAIN?
Do the ONE-ARMED KICKBACK described at bottom of page.

KICKBACK 2 WATER BOTTLES—ALL LEVELS

STARTING POSITION

- Feet shoulder width apart, knees slightly bent.
- Bend forward from hip until back is parallel—or just above parallel—to the floor.
- Elbows are bent at 90° angles, upper arms level with the back.

POSTURE: Abs tight, chest lifted, shoulders down and back, eyes straight ahead.

TIMING: 6 sec reps: 4 secs extending elbows, 2 secs return.

PROPER FORM

1 Exhale. Extend elbows until upper arms are parallel to floor.

2 Inhale. Bend elbows and return to SP.

3 Keep arms close to sides at all phases of motion.

COMMON MISTAKES

- *Rounding back.*
- *Elbows wandering from sides of body.*
- *Dropping elbows below level of back.*

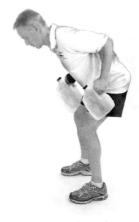
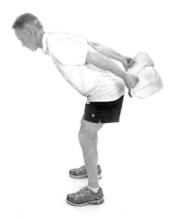

start/end position   *mid-point position*

INTERMEDIATE PROGRESSION
• Increase intensity by increasing weight.

ADVANCED BALANCE CHALLENGE
• Do exercise on one leg, change legs.

ONE-ARMED KICKBACK 1 WATER BOTTLE

Do this exercise if you have a history of lower back pain.

STARTING POSITION
• Kneel with right knee in center of a cushioned chair.
• Left leg is standing on floor, knee at same level as other knee and slightly bent.
• Right hand rests on chair directly under right shoulder.
• Elbow is bent at a 90° angle, upper arm is level with back.
• Follow form steps 1–3, change position and repeat with opposite arm

HISTORY OF LOWER BACK PAIN?
Change SP to sitting in a chair with back support. Follow form steps 1–2.

STANDING CURL 2 WATER BOTTLES—ALL LEVELS

STARTING POSITION

- Stand with feet shoulder width apart, knees slightly bent.
- Arms are extended at sides, palms facing up, each hand holds 1 WB.

POSTURE: Abs tight, chest lifted, shoulders down and back, eyes straight ahead.

TIMING: 6 sec reps: 2 secs up, 4 secs down.

PROPER FORM

1 Exhale. With elbows remaining close to body, raise WBs toward shoulders.

2 Inhale. Straighten elbows and return to SP.

COMMON MISTAKES

- *Shrugging shoulders; swinging upper body.*
- *Elbows wandering away from body.*

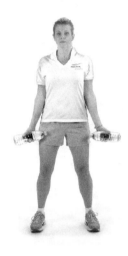
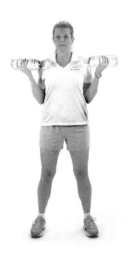

start/end position   *mid-point position*

INTERMEDIATE PROGRESSION
• Increase intensity by increasing weight.

ADVANCED BALANCE CHALLENGE: ALTERNATING ONE-LEGGED CURL
• Stand on one leg. Follow form steps 1–2, alternating arms, change legs and repeat.

VARIATION: HAMMER CURL
• To engage the forearms along with the biceps, change to a neutral grip with palms facing each other. Follow form steps 1–2.

HINT: Subtle difference between Standing Curl and Hammer Curl
Standing Curl = palms face up
Hammer Curl = palms face each other

COMBO
EXERCISES

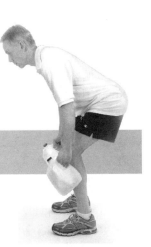

Combo
Exercises

These exercise combinations simultaneously work
the upper and lower body.

SQUAT/ROW COMBO 2 WBS—ADVANCED LEVEL

STARTING POSITION

- Feet shoulder width apart, toes straight ahead.
- Bend forward from hip until back is parallel—or just above parallel—
  to the floor.
- Knees are slightly bent, arms extended at sides, palms facing each
  other, each hand holds a WB.

POSTURE: Abs tight, chest lifted, shoulders down and back,
eyes straight ahead.

PROPER FORM

1 Bend knees and lower to squat position.
2 As you straighten knees, simultaneously bend elbows,
  bringing elbows even or beyond the level of the back.
3 Squat and lower WBs simultaneously.
4 Continue coordinated movement, breathing naturally.

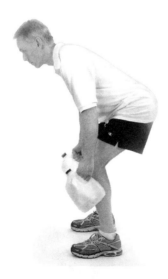

Movements require both coordination and concentration.
Their rhythmic nature increases heart rate while challenging several muscles at once.
Combination exercises are for Advanced Level ONLY.

SQUAT/SHOULDER PRESS COMBO 2 WBS—ADVANCED LEVEL

STARTING POSITION

- Stand with feet shoulder width apart, toes straight ahead.
- Arms form a 90° angle between elbow and shoulder.
- Palms face forward, holding WBs.

POSTURE: Abs tight, chest lifted, shoulders down and back, eyes straight ahead.

PROPER FORM

1 Bend knees and lower to squat position.

2 As you straighten knees, simultaneously straighten elbows.

3 Return elbows to SP as you begin to squat.

4 Continue coordinated movement, breathing naturally.

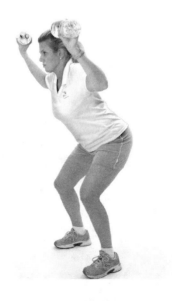

SQUAT/OVERHEAD EXTENSION COMBO 1 WB—ADVANCED LEVEL

STARTING POSITION

- Stand with feet shoulder width apart, toes straight ahead.
- Hands hold one WB overhead, fingers interlaced.
- Elbows are soft (not bent, not straight).

POSTURE: Abs tight, chest lifted, shoulders down and back, eyes straight ahead.

PROPER FORM

1 Bend knees until thighs are parallel to ground, while simultaneously bending elbows to form 90° angles.

2 Simultaneously straighten knees and elbows and return to SP.

3 Continue coordinated movement, breathing naturally.

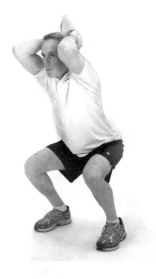

STARTING POSITION

- Stand with feet wider than shoulder width.
- Toes point at a 45° angle.
- Arms are extended at sides, palms facing up, each holds one WB.

POSTURE: Abs tight, chest lifted, shoulders down and back, eyes straight ahead.

PROPER FORM

1 Bend knees and elbows simultaneously as you lift WBs toward shoulders.

2 Simultaneously straighten elbows and knees as you return to SP.

3 Continue coordinated movement, breathing naturally.

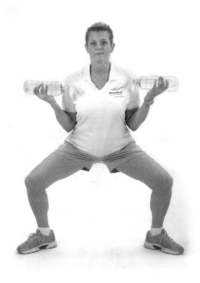

SQUAT/LATERAL RAISE COMBO 2 WBS—ADVANCED LEVEL

STARTING POSITION

- Stand with feet shoulder width apart.
- Arms are extended, palms face sides of thighs, each holds one WB.

POSTURE: Abs tight, chest lifted, shoulders down and back, eyes straight ahead.

PROPER FORM

1 As knees bend, simultaneously raise WBs to shoulder height.

2 Straighten knees and simultaneously lower arms.

3 Continue coordinated movement, breathing naturally.

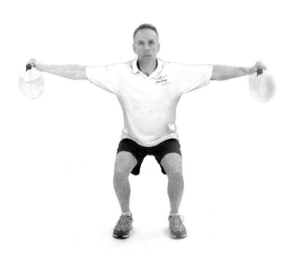

STARTING POSITION

- Stand with feet shoulder width apart.
- Left hand holds one WB, palm facing thigh, right arm is relaxed.

POSTURE: Abs tight, chest lifted, shoulders down and back, eyes straight ahead.

PROPER FORM

1 Take a long step forward with the left leg, bending each knee to a 90° angle.

2 Right heel is lifted, left knee over ankle.

3 As you bend knees, simultaneously bend the left elbow as you draw WB up until even with torso.

4 Simultaneously extend arm and straighten legs.

5 Continue coordinated movement, breathing naturally.

6 Change legs, hold WB in right hand. Follow form steps 1–5.

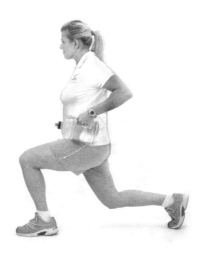

HAMMER CURL/TRAVELING LUNGE COMBO 2 WBS—ADVANCED LEVEL

STARTING POSITION

- Feet shoulder width apart.
- Arms are extended, palms facing sides of thighs, each holds one WB.

POSTURE: Abs tight, chest lifted, shoulders down and back, eyes straight ahead.

PROPER FORM

1 Step forward with left foot.

2 As you bend left knee, simultaneously bend both elbows and bring WBs toward shoulders.

3 Simultaneously straighten left knee and elbows as you step forward with the right foot.

4 Simultaneously bend both elbows and bring WBs toward shoulders.

5 Repeat coordinated movement, breathing naturally.

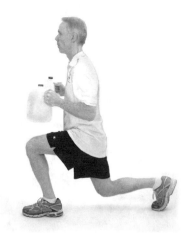

CORE
EXERCISES

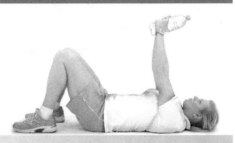

HISTORY OF NECK PAIN?
Eliminate Water Bottle. Support head with hands, elbows pointing out to sides. Do NOT interlace fingers. Follow form steps 1–3.

BASIC CRUNCH 1 WATER BOTTLE—ALL LEVELS

STARTING POSITION

- Lie on mat or cushioned floor, knees bent, feet shoulder width apart.
- Hold one WB above the chest, fingers interlaced for maximum weight support.
- Elbows are soft (not bent, not straight).

POSTURE: Abs tight, lower back on floor, shoulders down and back, eyes focused on ceiling.

TIMING: 6 sec reps: 2 secs up—pause—4 secs down.

PROPER FORM

1 Exhale. Contracting abs and looking at the ceiling, lift shoulder blades slightly off the floor.

2 Pause.

3 Inhale. Return to SP.

COMMON MISTAKES

- *Tucking chin, looking down.*
- *Raising shoulder blades too high.*

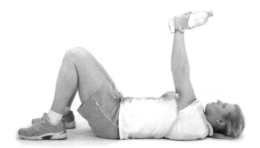
start/end position

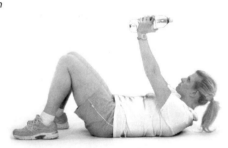
mid-point position

INTERMEDIATE PROGRESSION
• Increase intensity by increasing weight.

ADVANCED CHALLENGES
• To increase tension on abs, do not let shoulders touch floor between reps.

ALTERNATE KNEE WB CRUNCH
• As you lift shoulder blade, draw right knee toward WB. Pause. Return. Alternate knees.

HISTORY OF NECK PAIN?
Eliminate Water Bottle. Support head with hands, elbows pointing out to sides. Do NOT interlace fingers. Follow form steps 1–4.

OBLIQUE CRUNCH 1 WB—ALL LEVELS

STARTING POSITION

- Lie on mat or cushioned floor, knees bent, feet shoulder width apart.
- Hold one WB above the chest, fingers interlaced for maximum weight support.
- Elbows are soft (not bent, not straight).

POSTURE: Abs tight, lower back on floor, shoulders down and back, eyes focused on ceiling.

TIMING: 6 sec reps: 2 secs up—pause—4 secs down.

PROPER FORM

1 Exhale. Contracting abs and looking at the ceiling, lift shoulder blades slightly off the floor and bring WB toward left knee.
2 Pause.
3 Inhale. Return to SP.
4 Repeat steps 1–3 while moving WB toward right knee.

COMMON MISTAKES

- *Tucking chin; looking down.*
- *Twisting head from side to side.*

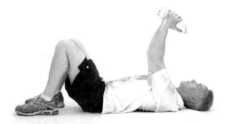

start/end position

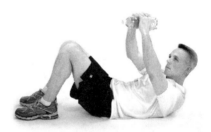

mid-point position

INTERMEDIATE PROGRESSION
- Increase intensity by increasing weight.

ADVANCED CHALLENGES
- To increase tension on abs, do not let shoulders touch floor between reps.

ALTERNATE KNEE WB OBLIQUE CRUNCH
- As you lift shoulder blades, draw right knee toward WB. Pause. Return. Alternate knees.

BRIDGE 1 WB—ALL LEVELS

STARTING POSITION

- Lie on mat or cushioned floor, knees bent, feet shoulder width apart.
- Hold one WB at center of abs, fingers interlaced for maximum weight support.
- Elbows are soft (not bent, not straight).

POSTURE: Abs tight, lower back on floor, shoulders down and back, eyes focused on ceiling.

TIMING: 6 sec reps: 2 secs up—pause—4 secs down.

PROPER FORM

1 Exhale. Contracting abs and buttocks, raise hips off floor until a straight line forms between hips and shoulders.

2 Pause.

3 Inhale. Return to SP.

COMMON MISTAKES

- *Lifting hips too high.*
- *Shrugging shoulders.*

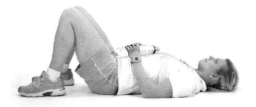

start/end position

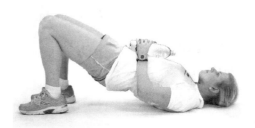

mid-point position

"GREEN" PLANK 2 STAINLESS STEEL WBS—ALL LEVELS

STARTING POSITION

- On a mat or cushioned floor, position stainless steel WBs shoulder width apart.
- Hold firmly onto WBs, elbows are soft (not bent, not straight).
- Knees are bent and resting on mat.

POSTURE: Abs and buttocks tight, head in line with spine, chin tucked.

TIMING: Hold for 1 minute. Relax.

PROPER FORM

1 Extend legs backward and lift body off floor until a straight line forms between head and feet.

2 Hold for 1 minute. Relax.

3 Breathe naturally throughout exercise.

COMMON MISTAKES

- *Letting hips sag.*
- *Shrugging shoulders.*
- *Lifting head.*

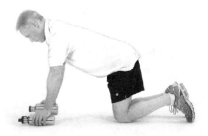

start/end position

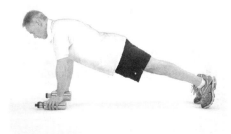

mid-point position

BEGINNERS
- Modify exercise by keeping knees in contact with floor while lifting hips. Hold for up to 1 minute, or as long as comfortable. Relax.

INTERMEDIATE/ADVANCED CHALLENGE:
ONE-LEGGED GREEN WB PLANK
- Lift one leg and hold plank form for one minute. Relax and change legs.

BIRD DOG 1 WB—ALL LEVELS

STARTING POSITION

- On a mat or cushioned floor, kneel and place right hand on floor under right shoulder.
- Left arm is extended in front of body, holding WB one inch above floor, palm facing floor.

POSTURE: Abs tight, back flat, head in line with spine.

TIMING: 6 sec reps. 2 secs lift—pause—4 secs return.

PROPER FORM

1 Exhale. Simultaneously raise left arm and extend right leg until parallel with floor.

2 Pause.

3 Inhale. Return to SP.

4 Slide WB to right hand and follow form steps 1–3.

5 Continue, alternating arms and legs.

COMMON MISTAKES

- *Lifting arm or leg too high.*
- *Rounding back.*
- *Lifting head.*

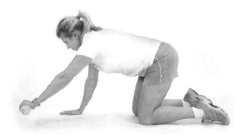

start/end position

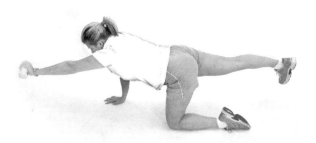

mid-point position

BEGINNERS

- Modify exercise by lying on stomach, both arms are extended in front of the body. Left hand holds WB, palm facing floor. Lift left arm and right leg simultaneously until parallel with floor. Pause and return to SP. Slide WB to right hand and repeat exercise, lifting left leg and right arm. Continue, alternating arms and legs.

INTERMEDIATE/ADVANCED CHALLENGE

- Slower speed—10 sec reps: 6 secs lift—pause—4 secs return.

TIME-EFFICIENT WORKOUTS

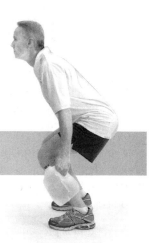

RULE OF THUMB: *you may go down a level, but never do a workout higher than your current ability.*

The following four workouts are carefully planned to challenge every level from beginner through advanced. Before attempting any of these workouts, familiarize yourself with all exercises in this book. When you are comfortable with the proper form of each exercise, choose the workout circuit that corresponds to your current fitness level (see Guidelines on pages v–viii).

If you are a beginner, never do an intermediate or advanced workout until you have mastered the beginner workout and feel the need for a greater challenge. If you are at the intermediate or advanced level and haven't worked out for a while, or desire a less strenuous workout on a particular day, you may elect to do an easier workout.

Each workout is presented as a circuit; the Advanced WB Workout has two circuits. Each circuit is a sequence of exercises designed to challenge those at a particular fitness level.

Always do circuits in the suggested order to gain maximum benefit.

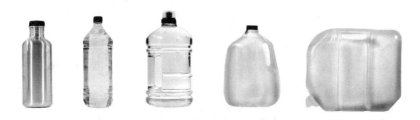

Once you progress past the beginner level, it is recommended that you alternate among the workouts at least every six weeks. This will prevent your muscles from adapting to a particular circuit, and help you to continue to make further strength gains.

BEGINNER WATER BOTTLE WORKOUT

These circuits utilize basic exercises that target a particular body part. The exercises progress from larger muscles to smaller ones, because larger muscles require more energy and are best addressed at the beginning of a workout when the body is fresh.

One set = 10–15 reps. Begin with 10 reps and work up to 15. Do only one set of each exercise.

There are two circuits in the Beginner WB Workout, each of which is a full-body challenge. The first month of your exercise program, do only Circuit #1. As your strength and endurance progress, you may elect to add Circuit #2. If only doing one circuit, always do Circuit #1.

REST PERIODS: 30 seconds between each exercise. Rest at least one minute between circuits, if doing both.

FREQUENCY: Twice a week, with at least 48 hours of rest between workouts. For example, workout on Monday and Thursday or Tuesday and Saturday.

Always warm up before working out and stretch afterwards.

BEGINNER WATER BOTTLE WORKOUT / CIRCUIT #1

Exercise	Reps	Sets	Page
Standard Squat	10–15	1	2
Chest Press	10–15	1	16
One-Armed Row	10–15	1	12
Seated Shoulder Press	10–15	1	22
One-Armed Kickback	10–15	1	33
Standing Curl	10–15	1	34
Basic Crunch	10–15	1	48
Bridge	0–15	1	52
Oblique Crunch	10–15	1	50
"Green" Plank (Beginners Modified)	Hold 30 secs		55

BEGINNER WATER BOTTLE WORKOUT / CIRCUIT #2

Exercise	Reps	Sets	Page
Plié Squat	10–15	1	4
Seated Row	10–15	1	10
Chest Fly	10–15	1	18
Lateral Raise	10–15	1	24
Overhead Extension	10–15	1	30
Hammer Curl	10–15	1	35
Basic Crunch	10–15	1	48
Bridge	10–15	1	52
Oblique Crunch	10–15	1	50
"Green" Plank (Beginners Modified)	Hold 30 secs		55

INTERMEDIATE WATER BOTTLE WORKOUT

These circuits again utilize basic exercises that target a particular body part, but the sequence is more challenging. Instead of progressing steadily from larger to smaller muscles line in the Beginner WB Circuits, these exercises alternate between muscles of the upper and lower body. Rest periods are shorter, frequency is greater and the volume of exercises is increased.

One set = 10–15 reps. Begin with 10 reps and work up to 15. Do only one set of each exercise.

There are two circuits in the Intermediate WB Workout, each of which is a full-body challenge. If only doing one circuit, always do Circuit #1. If time allows, you may add Circuit #2.

REST PERIODS: 15 secs (or less) between each exercise. Rest at least one minute between circuits.

FREQUENCY: Three times a week, with at least 24 hours of rest between workouts. For example, workout on Monday, Wednesday, Friday, or Tuesday, Thursday, Saturday.

Always warm up before working out and stretch afterwards.

INTERMEDIATE WATER BOTTLE WORKOUT / CIRCUIT #1

Exercise	Reps	Sets	Page
Standard Squat	10–15	1	2
Chest Press	10–15	1	16
Alternating Lunge	10–15	1	6
One-Armed Row	10–15	1	12
Deadlift	10–15	1	8
Seated Shoulder Press	10–15	1	22
Overhead Extension	10–15	1	30
Standing Curl	10–15	1	34
Basic Crunch	10–15	1	48
Bird Dog	10–15	1	56
Alternate Knee Oblique Crunch	10–15	1	51
"Green" Plank	Hold 45 secs		54
Oblique Crunch	10–15	1	50

INTERMEDIATE WATER BOTTLE WORKOUT / CIRCUIT #2

Exercise	Reps	Sets	Page
Plié Squat	10–15	1	4
Chest Fly	10–15	1	18
Alternating Lunge	10–15	1	6
One-Armed Row	10–15	1	12
Deadlift	10–15	1	8
Upright Row	10–15	1	26
Kickback	10–15	1	32
Hammer Curl	10–15	1	35
Basic Crunch (Alternate Knee WB Crunch)	10–15	1	49
"Green" Plank	10–15	1	54
Alternate Knee WB Oblique Crunch	10–15	1	51
Bird Dog	10–15	1	56

ADVANCED WATER BOTTLE WORKOUT

This is a challenging time-efficient workout for those wanting to increase their cardiovascular endurance and strength simultaneously. These circuits utilize exercises that combine upper and lower body movements. Cardiovascular intervals are interspersed between exercises. Rest periods are shorter.

There are two circuits in the Advanced WB Workout, each of which is a full-body challenge. If only doing one circuit, always do Circuit #1. If time allows, you may add Circuit #2.

One set = 10–15 reps. Begin with 10 reps and work up to 15. Do only one set of each exercise.

REST PERIODS: 10 secs (or less) between each exercise. Rest at least one minute between circuits.

FREQUENCY: Three times a week, with at least 24 hours of rest between workouts. For example, workout on Monday, Wednesday, Friday, or Tuesday, Thursday, Saturday.

Always warm up before working out and stretch afterwards.

CARDIO INTERVALS
During these 3 minute intervals, choose either jumping rope or shadow-boxing. Or combine them (e.g. 1 ½ minutes of each).

JUMPING ROPE
You may skip rope or, for a greater challenge, jump with both feet. If no rope is available, simulate movement and remember to move arms.

SHADOW-BOXING
Sparring with an imaginary opponent is both stimulating and fun. Keep feet in motion throughout.

 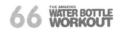

ADVANCED WATER BOTTLE WORKOUT / CIRCUIT #1

Exercise	Reps	Sets	Page
Squat-Row Combo	10–15	1	38
Chest Press	10–15	1	16
3 Minute Jump Rope/Boxing Interval			
Squat/Shoulder Press Combo	10–15	1	39
Squat/Overhead Extension Combo	10–15	1	40
3 Minute Jump Rope/Boxing Interval			
Plié Squat/Bicep Curl Combo	10–15	1	41
"Green" Plank	Hold 1 minute		54
Basic Crunch	10–15	1	48

ADVANCED WATER BOTTLE WORKOUT / CIRCUIT #2

Exercise	Reps	Sets	Page
Lunge/One-Armed Row Combo	10–15	1	43
Chest Fly	10–15	1	18
3 Minute Jump Rope/Boxing Interval			
Squat/Lateral Raise Combo	10–15	1	42
Squat/Overhead Extension Combo	10–15	1	40
3 Minute Jump Rope/Boxing Interval			
Hammer Curl/Traveling Lunge Combo	10–15	1	44
Bird Dog	10–15	1	56
Alternate Knee WB Oblique Crunch	10–15	1	51

TO MAKE A CIRCUIT EVEN MORE CHALLENGING, ALTERNATE CARDIO INTERVALS AFTER *EACH* EXERCISE.

LIGHTNING WATER BOTTLE WORKOUT—ALL LEVELS

This workout is most efficient for those who have limited time. If you wish to quickly challenge your entire body, you can do so with these eight exercises. The first four work the upper and lower body. The last four engage the core.

One set = 10–15 reps. Begin with 10 reps and work up to 15. Do only one set of each exercise.

There are two circuits in the Lightning WB Workout, each of which is a full-body challenge. If only doing one circuit, always do Circuit #1. If time allows, you may add Circuit #2.

REST PERIODS: 10–30 secs between each exercise, depending on your fitness level. Rest at least one minute between circuits.

Always warm up before working out and stretch afterwards.

LIGHTNING WATER BOTTLE WORKOUT / CIRCUIT #1

Exercise	Reps	Sets	Page
Standard Squat	10–15	1	2
Chest Press	10–15	1	16
Alternating Lunge	10–15	1	6
One-Armed Row	10–15	1	12
Basic Crunch	10–15	1	48
"Green" Plank	Hold 30 secs to 1 minute		54
Oblique Crunch	10–15	1	50
Bridge	10–15	1	52

LIGHTNING WATER BOTTLE WORKOUT / CIRCUIT #2

Exercise	Reps	Sets	Page
Plié Squat	10–15	1	4
Chest Fly	10–15	1	18
Deadlift	10–15	1	8
One-Armed Row	10–15	1	12
Bridge	10–15	1	52
Basic Crunch	10–15	1	48
"Green" Plank	Hold 30 secs to 1 minute		54
Bird Dog	10–15	1	56

BALANCE

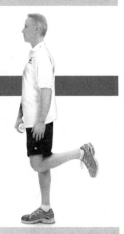

Everyone needs an intact balance system to accomplish everyday activities, such as getting out of a chair, climbing stairs or participating in sports.

Balance is defined in many ways. The National Academy of Sports Medicine defines balance as "The ability to sustain or return the body's center of mass or line of gravity over its base of support."

Balance diminishes with age. But any lack of activity can weaken muscles that ensure stability. The major components of balance are:

- postural alignment
- core strength
- strong thigh muscles
- ankle strength

Balance can be improved by practice at any age. To see an improvement in your stability, do the following postures 5–10 minutes a day. Begin by holding each posture for 10 seconds. Progress over time to 30 seconds, then minutes.

KEYS TO BALANCE PROGRESSIONS

- To help maintain the posture, focus on a point directly in front of you.
- If you have trouble balancing, hold a wall for support. Progress to less support (1 hand, then 2 fingers, 1 finger, then let go).
- Once you can easily balance in each posture, raise the WB for more of a challenge.
- Then try closing one eye.
- Then close both eyes.

CLOSE STANCE 1 WATER BOTTLE

STARTING POSITION

- Feet shoulder width apart.
- Right arm holds WB at side, palm toward thigh.

POSTURE: Abs tight, chest lifted, shoulders down and back, eyes straight ahead, focused on a single point.

PROPER FORM

1 Move left foot toward right foot until they touch.

2 Hold for 10 secs.

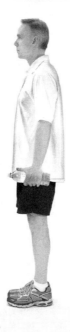

BALANCE PROGRESSION #1: Extend right arm and raise WB above head. Hold for 15 secs. Lower arm, change WB to left hand and raise. Hold for 15 secs.

BALANCE PROGRESSION #2: Repeat Balance Progression #1 while closing one eye. Hold for 20 secs.

BALANCE PROGRESSION #3: Repeat Balance Progression #1 while closing both eyes. Hold for 30 secs.

TOE-HEEL STANCE 1 WATER BOTTLE

STARTING POSITION

- Feet shoulder width apart.
- Left arm holds WB at side, palm toward thigh.

POSTURE: Abs tight, chest lifted, shoulders down and back, eyes straight ahead, focused on a single point.

PROPER FORM

1 Place left foot directly in front of right foot, back toe touches front heel. Hold for 10 secs.

2 Reverse foot placement and hold for 10 secs.

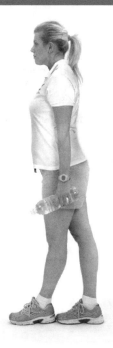

BALANCE PROGRESSION #1: With left foot in front, hold WB in left hand. Raise WB above head. Hold for 15 secs. Lower arm, change WB to right hand, reverse foot placement and raise WB. Hold for 15 secs.

BALANCE PROGRESSION #2: Repeat Balance Progression #1 while closing one eye. Hold for 20 secs.

BALANCE PROGRESSION #3: Repeat Balance Progression #1 while closing both eyes. Hold for 30 secs.

ONE-LEGGED STAND 1 WATER BOTTLE

STARTING POSITION

- Feet shoulder width apart.
- Right arm holds WB at front of leg, palm toward thigh.

POSTURE: Abs tight, chest lifted, shoulders down and back, eyes straight ahead, focused on a single point.

PROPER FORM

1 Bend left knee and raise foot off floor. Hold for 10 secs.

2 Change legs and repeat.

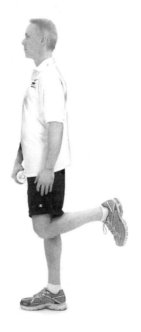

BALANCE PROGRESSION #1: Bend left knee and raise foot off floor. Keeping right arm straight, raise WB to shoulder height. Hold for 15 secs. Lower arm, change WB to left hand, reverse legs and raise WB. Hold for 15 secs.

BALANCE PROGRESSION #2: Repeat Balance Progression #1 while closing one eye. Hold for 20 secs.

BALANCE PROGRESSION #3: Repeat Balance Progression #1 while closing both eyes. Hold for 30 secs.

STRETCHES

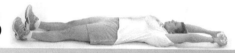

Stretching is an extremely important and often neglected part of any fitness program. If time permits, stretch after your warm-up. But you should always stretch after each workout.

WHY STRETCH?
When you exercise, muscles contract. Stretching returns muscles to their pre-workout length. Stretching also:

- increases overall ROM,
- reduces soreness after exercising,
- decreases risk of injury,
- improves posture.

KEYS TO STRETCHING
Stretch every day for 5–10 minutes.

- If stretching on non-workout days, always warm up for 5–10 minutes before stretching (see page vii).
- Do three reps of each stretch. Hold each rep 20–30 secs.
- Do not bounce.
- Maintain proper posture throughout stretch.
- Breathe naturally.

STARTING POSITION

- Kneel on a mat or cushioned floor.
- Extend arms in front, holding WB.

POSTURE: Shoulders relaxed, head in line with spine, eyes looking at floor.

PROPER FORM

1 Drop buttocks to heels.

2 Hold 20–30 secs.

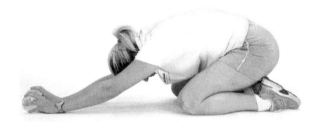

HAMSTRING STRETCH 2 WATER BOTTLES

STARTING POSITION

- Feet shoulder width apart.
- Arms extended, palms face sides of thighs, holding WBs.

POSTURE: Abs tight, chest lifted, shoulders down and back, eyes straight ahead.

PROPER FORM

1 Step forward with left leg, weight is on heel, toes off floor.

2 Right leg is slightly bent.

3 Lean forward from hip, body weight moves toward left leg, keep chest lifted.

4 Without rounding back, hold stretch for 20–30 secs.

5 Step back with left foot and repeat form steps 1–4 using right leg.

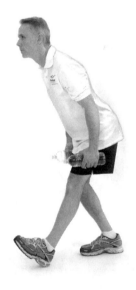

CALF STRETCH 1 WATER BOTTLE

STARTING POSITION

- Stand with feet shoulder width apart.
- Take a long step forward with left foot until back toe and front heel are lined up.
- With WB in left hand, extend WB overhead.

POSTURE: Abs tight, chest lifted, shoulders down and back, eyes straight ahead.

PROPER FORM

1 Keeping right leg straight and heel down, bend left knee as you lean forward from hip. Weight should move toward direction of front foot. Hold 20–30 secs.

2 Change legs and move WB to opposite hand. Repeat.

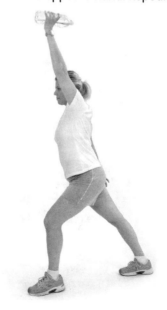

CAUTION! If you find balancing difficult in this posture, put WB down and hold wall for support.

QUAD STRETCH 1 WATER BOTTLE

STARTING POSITION

- Stand with feet shoulder width apart.
- With WB in left hand, extend left arm toward ceiling.

POSTURE: Abs tight, chest lifted, shoulders down and back, eyes straight ahead.

PROPER FORM

1 Bend right knee. Use right hand to draw foot toward right buttock.

2 Left knee is slightly bent.

3 Maintain posture throughout stretch. Hold for 20–30 secs.

4 Return to SP, changing WB to right hand.

5 Repeat form steps 1–3.

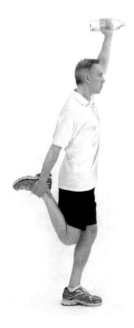

STARTING POSITION

- Lie on back on a mat or cushioned floor.
- Both arms are extended along floor behind head, holding WB.

POSTURE: Shoulders relaxed, lower back in contact with floor, eyes looking at ceiling.

PROPER FORM

1 Elongate body by simultaneously extending arms and legs.
2 Hold for 20–30 secs.

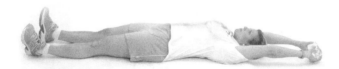

CHEST AND SHOULDER STRETCH 1 WATER BOTTLE

STARTING POSITION

- Feet shoulder width apart, knees soft (not bent, not straight).
- Arms are extended behind body holding WB.

POSTURE: Abs tight, chest lifted, shoulders down and back, eyes straight ahead.

PROPER FORM

1 Maintaining proper posture, raise WB to a comfortable position.

2 Hold 20–30 secs.

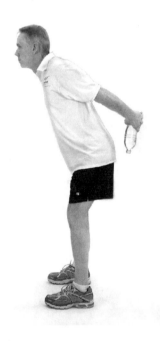